MARIJUANA EDIBLES COOKBOOK

Delicious Recipes for the Modern Cannabis Kitchen

Pedro D. Harlow

Table of Content

INTRODUCTION

In this unusual and tempting cookbook, i urge you to go on an investigation of tastes, doses, and the science behind cannabis-infused gastronomic pleasures.

This Marijuana Edibles Cookbook is a thorough handbook that exposes the secrets of producing magnificent foods that not only tempt the taste senses but also deliver a euphoric and therapeutic experience. Whether you are a seasoned cannabis enthusiast or an inquisitive epicurean, this book promises to be your trusted friend, presenting a harmonic combination of exquisite recipes and informative facts.

Chapter by chapter, I will dig into the wide universe of marijuana edibles, from grasping the complexities of dosage and portion management to mastering the art of crafting infused oils and butters. Delve into the intriguing science of cannabinoids and their interactions with the human body, giving you with a greater awareness of the plant's medical potential.

Beyond the kitchen, "marijuana edibles cookbook" also goes into the ever-evolving realm of marijuana politics, studying the historical backdrop of prohibition and the present landscape of legalization and social equality.

Whether you wish to upgrade your culinary talents, explore new gustatory frontiers, or just relish the joys of cannabis-infused products, this Marijuana Edibles Cookbook is your entrance to a tasty and educational experience. Get ready to excite your senses and learn the mysteries of this magical gastronomy universe. Let's begin this adventure together and raise our culinary experiences to new heights.

CHAPTER 1: INTRODUCTION TO MARIJUANA EDIBLES

Indulge in the mesmerizing world of marijuana sweets as we explore its delicious complexity. Discover numerous forms of edibles and how they interact with your body's endocannabinoid system. This chapter lays the setting for an informative voyage into the delightful world of cannabis-infused gastronomy.

Understanding Marijuana Edibles: An Overview

Marijuana edibles have evolved as a popular and intriguing alternative to conventional means of cannabis intake. This comprehensive overview unravels the mysteries behind these delectable treats, shedding light on their unique characteristics and effects.

Unlike smoking or vaping, edibles offer a discreet and smoke-free experience, making them appealing to a wide range of users. From delectable baked goods to savory delights, the diversity of edible options is vast, catering to varying taste preferences.

However, edibles require a nuanced understanding of dosing and onset times. The delayed onset of effects demands patience and caution to avoid overconsumption, as the potency can catch even experienced users off-guard.

In this chapter, we delve into the metabolism of cannabinoids when ingested, revealing how they transform in the body and influence the user's experience. We explore the importance of starting with a low dose, especially for beginners, and the significance of waiting for the effects to manifest fully.

Whether you're a novice or a seasoned enthusiast, this review offers you with vital information to explore the tempting world of marijuana sweets with confidence and curiosity.

Different Types of Edibles and Their Effects

Marijuana edibles provide a fascinating diversity of possibilities, each giving a distinct flavor and sensation. This thorough examination dives into the vast universe of food things, from sweet confections to savory treats, and the different sensations they produce.

Sweet Treats: Gourmet chocolates, scrumptious candies, and gorgeous brownies are just a few samples of the luxurious sweet delicacies available. These snacks generally take longer to kick in but deliver a longer-lasting and strong high.

Savory Delights: For individuals with a predilection for savory tastes, cannabis-infused foods like crackers, chips, and popcorn provide a tasty alternative. Savory edibles frequently have lower THC amounts, delivering a softer effect.

Beverages: Cannabis-infused drinks, including teas, sodas, and coffees, give a delightful way to ingest cannabinoids. Their effects might vary based on the beverage's intensity and the individual's tolerance.

Balanced Ratios: Some edibles have balanced ratios of THC and CBD, delivering a more balanced and therapeutic experience. These items are gaining popularity for their possible therapeutic effects.

Understanding the many kinds of edibles and their effects allows consumers to pick the choice that best matches with their tastes and intended experience. As with any cannabis usage, moderation and appropriate use are important to a safe and happy voyage into the realm of marijuana-infused pleasures.

Safety Precautions and Responsible Consumption

While marijuana edibles give a delightful and intriguing way to experience cannabis, cautious intake is crucial to guarantee a safe and happy experience. This thorough guide focuses on critical safety concerns and best practices for individuals stepping into the realm of cannabis-infused delights.

Dosing Awareness: Start with a minimal dosage, particularly for novices, and wait for at least 1 to 2 hours before contemplating further intake. The effects of edibles might be delayed, and overconsumption can lead to undesired and extreme sensations.

Label Reading: Always read the product labels to understand the strength of the consumable and the suggested serving amount. This information is critical for effective dosage and portion management.

Secure Storage: Keep marijuana edibles out of reach of children and pets, and keep them in a secure, marked container to prevent accidental consumption.

Clear Communication: If sharing edibles with others, describe the strength and possible consequences properly to ensure appropriate usage among friends and visitors.

Avoid Mixing with Alcohol or Drugs: Combining edibles with alcohol or other drugs may enhance the effects and raise the risk of unpleasant responses.

Understanding Personal Tolerance: Everyone's tolerance to cannabis varies, so be careful of individual variances and responses.

By following these safety measures and adopting responsible use, consumers may taste the joys of marijuana edibles with confidence, assuring a good and joyful experience while emphasizing their well-being.

The Endocannabinoid System and How Edibles Interact with It

The endocannabinoid system (ECS) plays a vital function in regulating different physiological processes in the human body. Comprising receptors, endocannabinoids, and enzymes, the ECS helps maintain homeostasis and equilibrium.

When ingesting marijuana edibles, cannabinoids like THC and CBD interact with the ECS. THC connects with the CB1 receptors largely present in the brain and central nervous system, resulting to psychoactive effects. On the other hand, CBD interacts with CB1 and CB2 receptors, impacting multiple systems, but without inducing intoxication.

Once consumed, the cannabinoids in edibles are processed in the liver, turning THC into its more powerful form, 11-hydroxy-THC. This mechanism leads to the delayed onset of effects and the possibly longer-lasting high experienced with edibles.

The ECS's participation in different biological processes, such as pain perception, mood control, and immunological response, helps explain the possible therapeutic benefits of marijuana edibles.

Understanding the relationship between cannabis and the endocannabinoid system sheds insight on the significant influence these tasty delights may have on our well-being. However, cautious usage and dose knowledge remain important to exploiting the medicinal potential of marijuana edibles efficiently.

CHAPTER 2: DOSAGE AND PORTION CONTROL

Mastering the art of dosage and portion control is key for a safe and pleasurable voyage into the realm of marijuana edibles. In this chapter, I uncover the subtleties of selecting the proper dose, recognizing its effects on individual experiences, and adopting effective portion control tactics. From novices to seasoned lovers, this comprehensive book gives you with the knowledge to traverse the domain of edibles with confidence and accuracy.

Importance of Accurate Dosage

The significance of appropriate marijuana edibles dosage cannot be emphasized, since it directly effects the user's experience and well-being. Overconsumption of edibles may lead to negative symptoms, such as anxiety, paranoia, and dizziness.

Unlike other ingestion techniques, edibles have a delayed start of effects, making it easy to misjudge their strength and mistakenly eat more.

Understanding and sticking to correct dose standards is vital to guarantee a regulated and pleasurable experience, enabling consumers to relish the advantages of cannabis-infused foods without the danger of overwhelming adverse effects. Responsible dosage helps folks to explore the world of edibles with confidence and awareness.

Factors Affecting Edible Dosage

Tolerance: Regular cannabis users often acquire a tolerance to cannabinoids, needing greater doses to produce the desired effects. Beginners or persons with poor tolerance levels should start with smaller dosages to prevent overconsumption.

Body Weight: Body weight may impact how cannabinoids are distributed and metabolized in the body. Generally, persons with greater body weight may need somewhat larger doses compared to those with lower body weight.

Experience: Previous experience with cannabis might impact how people react to edibles. Seasoned users could take bigger dosages more efficiently, but beginners should continue with care.

Metabolism: Variations in metabolism may alter how rapidly cannabinoids are absorbed and digested, affecting the onset and duration of effects.

Individual Sensitivity: Each person's biological chemistry is distinct, resulting to varied sensitivities to cannabinoids.

Considering these criteria helps consumers to tune their marijuana edible dose for a tailored and balanced experience, increasing the benefits while reducing any unwanted effects. Responsible dosage is important to unleashing the full potential of cannabis-infused food safely and efficiently.

Calculating Dosage: A Step-by-Step Guide

Calculating marijuana edibles dose takes accuracy and awareness to guarantee a regulated and satisfying experience. This step-by-step method gives a path for calculating the right dosage:

Know the THC Content: Check the THC content of the edible product, often mentioned on the package.

Divide THC Content: Divide the total THC content by the number of servings in the package to find the THC per serving.

Start Modest: For novices, begin with a modest dose, often 2.5-5mg of THC, to measure individual tolerance.

Monitor Effects: Wait for at least 1-2 hours after ingestion to analyze the effects before contemplating more dosages.

Gradual Raise: If required, gradually raise the dose in tiny increments to attain the perfect balance.

By following this guidance and being attentive of individual circumstances, users may confidently and properly enjoy the delights of marijuana edibles.

Portion Control Techniques: Ensuring Consistent Experience

Portion management is a vital part of ingesting marijuana edibles to guarantee a consistent and satisfying experience. These approaches assist consumers retain a feeling of balance and prevent overconsumption:

Divide the Edible: Cut or break the edible into smaller bits to manage dose precisely.

Label and keep: Label each piece with its THC concentration to avoid confusion and keep them properly to prevent unintentional overindulgence.

Journaling: Keep a log of eaten portions and their effects to monitor individual reactions and adjust future dosages appropriately.

Wait for Effects: Allow adequate time between portions to analyze the effects before taking more.

By adopting these portion control tactics, users may maximize their edible experience, appreciating the benefits of cannabis while maintaining a conscious and responsible attitude to intake.

CHAPTER 3: CREATING MASTER INGREDIENTS

Unlock the secrets of making cannabis-infused oils and butters in this instructive chapter. Discover the art of decarboxylation, the process that activates the cannabinoids, and discover the step-by-step processes for infusing oils and butters with the benefits of marijuana. From exact measures to flavor-enhancing ideas, this chapter gives you with the fundamental skills to produce master ingredients that will lift your culinary adventures to new heights of enjoyment.

Decarboxylation: Activating Cannabinoids for Infusion

Decarboxylation is a vital procedure in preparing cannabis for infusion into oils and butters used in marijuana edibles. This transformational phase includes applying heat to raw cannabis flower or trim to convert the inactive acidic cannabinoids (THCA and CBDA) into its active counterparts (THC and CBD). Without decarboxylation, the edibles would lack the required euphoric and medicinal properties.

The technique operates by removing a carboxyl group from the cannabis molecules with the use of heat. This technique is best done at temperatures between 200°F to 240°F (93°C to 115°C) for a set length, often about 30 to 45 minutes. Overheating or extended exposure may lead to cannabinoid breakdown, decreasing the strength and taste of the final product.

Decarboxylation is a critical step for making consistent and dependable cannabis-infused oils and butters. It guarantees that the required strength and effects are obtained in the final product, enabling consumers to experience the full potential of cannabis while taking the edibles.

By mastering the technique of decarboxylation, cannabis fans may unlock the actual power of the plant's components and raise their culinary creations to new heights of quality and effectiveness. Whether producing savory meals or sweet pastries, knowing the chemistry underlying decarboxylation helps chefs to boldly blend their master ingredients with the medicinal benefits of cannabis.

Measuring Potency

Measuring the strength of cannabis is vital for attaining consistent results when infusing oils and butters for marijuana edibles. The two principal cannabinoids of relevance are THC (tetrahydrocannabinol) and CBD (cannabidiol), each presenting various affects and advantages.

Potency testing entails detecting the levels of THC and CBD in the cannabis used for infusion. This information enables chefs to compute the precise quantity of THC contained in the final product, allowing proper dosage and portion management.

Laboratories equipped with advanced analytical methods, such as high-performance liquid chromatography (HPLC) or gas chromatography (GC), are employed to detect cannabis levels accurately. The findings are generally stated as a percentage of THC or CBD by weight.

Understanding the strength of cannabis used in infusion is crucial for various reasons. It permits consumers to customise edibles to their desired effects, whether wanting a light or more intense experience. Moreover, it assists in maintaining uniformity among batches, delivering a predictable and satisfying output.

By appreciating the importance of detecting THC and CBD levels, cooks may fine-tune their recipes, ensuring that each infused food provides the ideal benefits. With this information, marijuana edibles can be produced with precision and confidence, giving cunsumers an amazing and individualized gastronomic voyage into the realm of cannabis-infused delicacies.

Tips & Tricks for Flavorful Infusions

Creating cannabis-infused oils and butters not only entails understanding the science of decarboxylation and calculating potency but also needs attention to the art of taste infusion. Enhancing the flavor of infused substances is key to making tasty and attractive marijuana edibles. Here are some suggestions and strategies to produce tasty infusions:

Select Quality Cannabis: Start with high-quality cannabis flower or trim with rich terpene profiles, since terpenes add to the overall taste of the infusion.

Strain Selection: Different cannabis strains give a broad spectrum of tastes, from fruity to earthy to peppery. Experiment with strains to discover the ones that best suit your dish.

Low Heat Infusion: To retain delicate tastes and avoid a grassy taste, infuse oils and butters at low heat (below the boiling point) for a lengthy duration.

Aromatics: Enhance the infusion with aromatics like garlic, herbs, or citrus peels, giving depth and richness to the finished result.

Straining Method: After infusing, strain the liquid using fine mesh or cheesecloth to eliminate plant particles and retain a smooth consistency.

Storage and Shelf Life: Store infused oils and butters in sealed containers in a cold, dark area to maintain their tastes and potency.

Dose Balance: Ensure that the infused ingredient's strength matches the recipe's total dose to ensure a consistent and satisfying experience.

By combining these ideas and tactics, chefs may improve the tastes of their cannabis-infused foods, making them into delectable culinary components. Whether crafting savory meals or sweet confections, flavorful infusions improve the attractiveness of marijuana edibles, making them a delightful and intriguing treat for all palates.

Marijuana edibles Sweet snacks Recipes

Recipe 1: Cannabis-Infused Gourmet Chocolates
Ingredients:

- 1 cup cannabis-infused coconut oil (made with decarboxylated cannabis and coconut oil)
- 1 cup unsweetened cocoa powder
- 1/4 cup honey or maple syrup
- 1 tsp vanilla extract
- Pinch of salt

Instructions for Creating Cannabis-Infused Coconut Oil:

- Decarboxylate 7-10 grams of finely powdered cannabis at 220°F (104°C) for 30-45 minutes.

- In a saucepan, slowly heat 1 cup of coconut oil over low heat.

- Add the decarboxylated cannabis to the coconut oil and mix.

- Simmer on low heat for 2-3 hours, stirring periodically.

- Strain the mixture through a strainer to remove plant detritus and store the infused coconut oil in a jar.

Instructions for Gourmet Chocolates:

- In a bowl, combine the cannabis-infused coconut oil, unsweetened cocoa powder, honey or maple syrup, vanilla essence, and a sprinkle of salt.

- Pour the mixture into chocolate molds or an ice cube tray.

- Place in the refrigerator for 1-2 hours or until the chocolates firm.

- Once firm, remove from the molds, and enjoy!

Dosage & Portion:

- Start with one chocolate containing around 5mg of THC.
- Wait for at least 1 hour before contemplating further intake.
- Adjust the dose in successive batches to fit individual tolerance levels.

Recipe 2: Cannabis-Infused Gummies

Ingredients:

- 1/2 cup cannabis-infused simple syrup (made with decarboxylated cannabis and a 1:1 mix of water and sugar)
- 1/2 cup fruit juice (e.g., orange, cherry, or raspberry)
- 3 tbsp unflavored gelatin Gummy molds

Instructions for Creating Cannabis-Infused Simple Syrup:

- Decarboxylate 7-10 grams of finely powdered cannabis at 220°F (104°C) for 30-45 minutes.
- In a saucepan, add 1 cup of water and 1 cup of sugar.
- Add the decarboxylated cannabis to the mixture and boil on low heat for 2-3 hours, stirring periodically.
- Strain the mixture through a strainer to remove plant detritus and store the infused simple syrup in a jar.

Instructions for Gummies:
- In a saucepan, cook the fruit juice over low heat.
- Add the cannabis-infused simple syrup and unflavored gelatin, stirring until totally dissolved.
- Pour the mixture into gummy molds.
- Refrigerate for 1-2 hours or until the gummies harden.

- Pop the gummies out of the molds and store in an airtight container.

Dosage & Portion:

- Start with one gummy containing around 5mg of THC.
- Wait for at least 1 hour before contemplating further intake.
- Adjust the dose in successive batches to fit individual tolerance levels.

Recipe 3: Cannabis-Infused Brownies

Ingredients:

- 1 cup cannabis-infused butter (made with decarboxylated cannabis and unsalted butter)
- 1 cup granulated sugar
- 1/2 cup unsweetened cocoa powder
- 2 big eggs
- 1 tsp vanilla extract
- 1/2 cup all-purpose flour
- 1/4 tsp baking powder
- Pinch of salt

- Optional: 1/2 cup chopped walnuts or chocolate chips

Instructions for Creating Cannabis-Infused Butter:

- Decarboxylate 7-10 grams of finely powdered cannabis at 220°F (104°C) for 30-45 minutes.
- In a saucepan, melt 1 cup of unsalted butter over low heat.
- Add the decarboxylated cannabis to the melted butter and boil on low heat for 2-3 hours, stirring periodically.
- Strain the mixture through a strainer to remove plant detritus and store the infused butter in a jar.

Instructions for Brownies:

- Preheat the oven to 350°F (175°C) and butter an 8x8-inch baking pan.
- In a mixing dish, combine the cannabis-infused butter, granulated sugar, and cocoa powder until completely combined.

- Beat in the eggs and vanilla extract.
- In a second basin, mix together the all-purpose flour, baking powder, and salt.
- Gradually add the dry ingredients to the wet components, stirring until just blended.
- Optionally, mix in chopped walnuts or chocolate chips.
- Pour the batter into the prepared baking pan and distribute it evenly.
- Bake for 20-25 minutes or until a toothpick inserted in the middle comes out with a few wet crumbs.
- Allow the brownies to cool before cutting into squares.

Dosage & Portion:
- Start with one brownie containing around 10mg of THC.
- Wait for at least 1 hour before contemplating further intake.
- Adjust the dose in successive batches to fit individual tolerance levels.

Recipe 4: Cannabis-Infused Lemon Bars

Ingredients:

- 1 cup cannabis-infused butter (made with decarboxylated cannabis and unsalted butter)
- 2 cups all-purpose flour
- 1/2 cup powdered sugar
- Pinch of salt
- 4 big eggs
- 1 1/2 cups granulated sugar
- 1/4 cup fresh lemon juice
- 1 tbsp lemon zest

Instructions for Creating Cannabis-Infused Butter:

- Decarboxylate 7-10 grams of finely powdered cannabis at 220°F (104°C) for 30-45 minutes.
- In a saucepan, melt 1 cup of unsalted butter over low heat.

- Add the decarboxylated cannabis to the melted butter and boil on low heat for 2-3 hours, stirring periodically.
- Strain the mixture through a strainer to remove plant detritus and store the infused butter in a jar.

Instructions for Lemon Bars:

- Preheat the oven to 350°F (175°C) and butter a 9x13-inch baking pan.
- In a mixing bowl, add 2 cups of all-purpose flour, powdered sugar, and a sprinkle of salt.
- Cut in 1/2 cup of cannabis-infused butter until the mixture resembles coarse crumbs.
- Press the mixture into the bottom of the prepared baking pan.
- Bake for 15-20 minutes or until gently browned.
- In a separate dish, mix together the eggs, granulated sugar, fresh lemon juice, and lemon zest.

- Pour the lemon mixture over the cooked crust.
- Bake for a further 20-25 minutes or until the lemon mixture is set.
- Allow the lemon bars to cool before cutting into squares.

Dosage & Portion:
- Start with one lemon bar containing around 10mg of THC.
- Wait for at least 1 hour before contemplating further intake.
- Adjust the dose in successive batches to fit individual tolerance levels.

Recipe 5: Cannabis-Infused Raspberry Thumbprint Cookies

Ingredients:

- 1 cup cannabis-infused butter (made with decarboxylated cannabis and unsalted butter)
- 1/2 cup granulated sugar
- 2 cups all-purpose flour
- 1/2 tsp vanilla extract
- 1/4 tsp salt
- 1/2 cup raspberry jam

Instructions for Creating Cannabis-Infused Butter:

- Decarboxylate 7-10 grams of finely powdered cannabis at 220°F (104°C) for 30-45 minutes.
- In a saucepan, melt 1 cup of unsalted butter over low heat.
- Add the decarboxylated cannabis to the melted butter and boil on low heat for 2-3 hours, stirring periodically.

- Strain the mixture through a strainer to remove plant detritus and store the infused butter in a jar.

Instructions for Raspberry Thumbprint Cookies:

- Preheat the oven to 375°F (190°C) and line a baking sheet with parchment paper.
- In a mixing bowl, cream together the cannabis-infused butter and granulated sugar until light and fluffy.
- Beat in the vanilla essence and salt.
- Gradually add the all-purpose flour, mixing until the dough comes together.
- Roll the dough into 1-inch balls and set them on the prepared baking sheet.
- Create a thumbprint indentation in the middle of each cookie.
- Fill each indentation with a dab of raspberry jam.
- Bake for 12-15 minutes or until the edges of the cookies are gently brown.

- Allow the cookies to cool on the baking pan before serving.

Dosage & Portion:

- Start with one cookie containing around 5mg of THC.
- Wait for at least 1 hour before contemplating further intake.
- Adjust the dose in successive batches to fit individual tolerance levels.

Savory Delight Recipes

Recipe 1: Cannabis-Infused Garlic Herb Butter
Ingredients:

- 1 cup cannabis-infused butter (made with decarboxylated cannabis and unsalted butter)
- 4 cloves garlic, minced
- 1 tbsp fresh parsley, freshly chopped
- 1 tbsp fresh thyme, freshly chopped
- 1/2 tsp salt
- 1/4 tsp black pepper

Instructions for Creating Cannabis-Infused Butter:

- Decarboxylate 7-10 grams of finely powdered cannabis at 220°F (104°C) for 30-45 minutes.

- In a saucepan, melt 1 cup of unsalted butter over low heat.

- Add the decarboxylated cannabis to the melted butter and boil on low heat for 2-3 hours, stirring periodically.

- Strain the mixture through a strainer to remove plant detritus and store the infused butter in a jar.

Instructions for Garlic Herb Butter:

- In a mixing bowl, combine the cannabis-infused butter, minced garlic, fresh parsley, fresh thyme, salt, and black pepper.

- Mix until all the ingredients are completely combined.

- Transfer the butter mixture to a piece of parchment paper or plastic wrap.

- Roll it into a log form and twist the ends to seal.
- Refrigerate until hard.
- Slice the infused butter and use it to lend a delicious edge to grilled meats, veggies, or toasted bread.

Dosage & Portion:
- Start with 1 spoonful of cannabis-infused butter containing roughly 10mg of THC.
- Wait for at least 1 hour before contemplating further intake.
- Adjust the dose in successive batches to fit individual tolerance levels.
- Recipe 2: Cannabis-Infused Roasted Vegetable Medley

Ingredients:
- 2 cups mixed veggies (e.g., carrots, bell peppers, zucchini, and cherry tomatoes)

- 2 tbsp cannabis-infused olive oil (made with decarboxylated cannabis and extra virgin olive oil)
- 1 tsp dried oregano
- 1 tsp dried thyme
- 1/2 tsp garlic powder
- Salt and black pepper to taste

Instructions for Creating Cannabis-Infused Olive Oil:

- Decarboxylate 7-10 grams of finely powdered cannabis at 220°F (104°C) for 30-45 minutes.
- In a saucepan, gradually heat 1 cup of extra virgin olive oil over low heat.
- Add the decarboxylated cannabis to the olive oil and mix.
- Simmer on low heat for 2-3 hours, stirring periodically.
- Strain the mixture through a strainer to remove plant detritus and store the infused olive oil in a jar.

Instructions for Roasted Vegetable Medley:

- Preheat the oven to 400°F (200°C) and line a baking sheet with parchment paper.
- In a bowl, combine the mixed veggies with the cannabis-infused olive oil, dried oregano, dried thyme, garlic powder, salt, and black pepper until equally coated.
- Spread the veggies on the prepared baking sheet in a single layer.
- Roast in the preheated oven for 20-25 minutes or until the veggies are soft and faintly browned.
- Serve the roasted veggie medley as a tasty and savory side dish.

Dosage & Portion:

- Start with one plate of roasted veggies containing around 5mg of THC.
- Wait for at least 1 hour before contemplating further intake.
- Adjust the dose in successive batches to fit individual tolerance levels.

Recipe 3: Cannabis-Infused Pesto Pasta

Ingredients:

- 1 cup fresh basil leaves
- 1/4 cup pine nuts
- 1/4 cup grated Parmesan cheese
- 2 cloves garlic
- 1/2 cup cannabis-infused olive oil (made with decarboxylated cannabis and extra virgin olive oil)
- Salt and black pepper to taste
- 8 oz pasta of your choice

Instructions for Pesto Pasta:

- In a food processor, mix the fresh basil leaves, pine nuts, grated Parmesan cheese, and garlic.
- Pulse until the ingredients are coarsely minced.
- With the food processor running, carefully sprinkle in the cannabis-infused olive oil until the pesto reaches your preferred consistency.

- Season with salt and black pepper to taste.
- Cook the pasta according to package directions, drain, and combine with the cannabis-infused pesto.
- Serve immediately, garnished with more grated Parmesan cheese if preferred.

Dosage & Portion:
- Start with one dish of cannabis-infused pesto pasta containing about 5mg of THC.
- Wait for at least 1 hour before contemplating further intake.
- Adjust the dose in successive batches to fit individual tolerance levels.

Recipe 4: Cannabis-Infused Herbed Focaccia Bread

Ingredients:
- 2 cups all-purpose flour
- 1 tsp active dry yeast
- 1 cup warm water

- 1/4 cup cannabis-infused olive oil (made with decarboxylated cannabis and extra virgin olive oil)
- 1 tsp dried rosemary
- 1 tsp dried thyme
- 1 tsp dried oregano
- 1/2 tsp garlic powder
- 1/2 tsp salt

Instructions for Herbed Focaccia Bread:

- In a large mixing bowl, add the all-purpose flour, active dry yeast, warm water, cannabis-infused olive oil, dried rosemary, dried thyme, dried oregano, garlic powder, and salt.
- Mix until a dough forms.
- Knead the dough on a floured surface for approximately 5-7 minutes until smooth and elastic.
- area the dough in a greased basin, cover with a wet towel, and let it rest in a warm area for 1-2 hours or until doubled in size.

- Preheat the oven to 425°F (220°C) and butter a baking sheet.
- Press the rising dough onto the baking sheet, forming a rectangle shape.
- Drizzle extra cannabis-infused olive oil over the dough and use your fingers to form indentations.
- Bake in the preheated oven for 20-25 minutes or until the focaccia is golden brown.
- Allow the herbed focaccia bread to cool slightly before slicing and serving.

Dosage & Portion:
- Start with one plate of herbed focaccia bread containing around 5mg of THC.
- Wait for at least 1 hour before contemplating further intake.
- Adjust the dose in successive batches to fit individual tolerance levels.

Recipe 5: Cannabis-Infused Stuffed Mushrooms

Ingredients:

- 12 big mushrooms, stems removed and conserved
- 1/2 cup cannabis-infused breadcrumbs (made with decarboxylated cannabis and store-bought breadcrumbs)
- 1/4 cup grated Parmesan cheese
- 2 cloves garlic, minced
- 2 tbsp fresh parsley, freshly chopped
- 1/4 cup cannabis-infused olive oil (made with decarboxylated cannabis and extra virgin olive oil)
- Salt and black pepper to taste

Instructions for Creating Cannabis-Infused Breadcrumbs:

- Decarboxylate 7-10 grams of finely powdered cannabis at 220°F (104°C) for 30-45 minutes.
- Mix the decarboxylated cannabis with store-bought breadcrumbs until fully blended.

- Store the cannabis-infused breadcrumbs in an airtight container.

Instructions for Stuffed Mushrooms:

- Preheat the oven to 375°F (190°C) and line a baking sheet with parchment paper.
- In a bowl, add the cannabis-infused breadcrumbs, grated Parmesan cheese, chopped garlic, fresh parsley, cannabis-infused olive oil, salt, and black pepper.
- Use a spoon to load each mushroom cap with the breadcrumb mixture, compressing it securely.
- Place the filled mushrooms on the prepared baking sheet.
- Bake in the preheated oven for 20-25 minutes or until the mushrooms are soft and the breadcrumbs are golden brown.
- Serve the cannabis-infused stuffed mushrooms as a tasty appetizer or side dish.

Dosage & Portion:

- Start with one serving of cannabis-infused stuffed mushrooms containing about 5mg of THC.

- Wait for at least 1 hour before contemplating further intake.

- Adjust the dose in successive batches to fit individual tolerance levels.

Marijuana Edibles Beverage Recipes

Recipe 1: Cannabis-Infused Classic Brownie Hot Chocolate

Ingredients:

- 2 cups whole milk
- 1/2 cup cannabis-infused chocolate syrup (made with decarboxylated cannabis and chocolate syrup)
- 1/4 cup unsweetened cocoa powder
- 1/4 cup granulated sugar
- 1/2 tsp vanilla extract

- Whipped cream with chocolate shavings for garnish

Instructions for Creating Cannabis-Infused Chocolate Syrup:

- Decarboxylate 7-10 grams of finely powdered cannabis at 220°F (104°C) for 30-45 minutes.
- In a saucepan, slowly cook 1 cup of chocolate syrup over low heat.
- Add the decarboxylated cannabis to the chocolate syrup and mix.
- Simmer on low heat for 1-2 hours, stirring periodically.
- Strain the mixture through a strainer to remove plant detritus and store the infused chocolate syrup in a jar.

Instructions for Brownie Hot Chocolate:

- In a saucepan, stir together the whole milk, cannabis-infused chocolate syrup, unsweetened cocoa powder, granulated sugar, and vanilla extract over medium heat.

- Heat until the mixture is heated but not boiling, stirring frequently.
- Remove from heat and pour the hot chocolate into cups.
- Top with whipped cream and chocolate shavings for a luscious finishing touch.

Dosage & Portion:

- Start with one cup of brownie hot chocolate containing roughly 10mg of THC.
- Wait for at least 1 hour before contemplating further intake.
- Adjust the dose in successive batches to fit individual tolerance levels.

Recipe 2: Cannabis-Infused Iced Chai Latte

Ingredients:

- 2 cups brewed chai tea, cooled
- 1 cup milk of your choice (e.g., almond, soy, or dairy)

- 1/4 cup cannabis-infused honey (made with decarboxylated cannabis and honey)
- 1 tsp vanilla extract
- Ice cubes

Instructions for Creating Cannabis-Infused Honey:

- Decarboxylate 7-10 grams of finely powdered cannabis at 220°F (104°C) for 30-45 minutes.
- In a saucepan, slowly cook 1 cup of honey over low heat.
- Add the decarboxylated cannabis to the honey and mix.
- Simmer on low heat for 1-2 hours, stirring periodically.
- Strain the mixture through a strainer to remove plant detritus and store the infused honey in a jar.

Instructions for Iced Chai Latte:

- In a pitcher, mix the cooled brewed chai tea, milk, cannabis-infused honey, and vanilla essence.

- Stir until properly blended and the honey is entirely dissolved.

- Fill glasses with ice cubes and pour the chai latte mixture over the ice.

- Stir gently and finish with a dusting of cinnamon if preferred.

Dosage & Portion:

- Start with one glass of iced chai latte containing around 5mg of THC.

- Wait for at least 1 hour before contemplating further intake.

- Adjust the dose in successive batches to fit individual tolerance levels.

Recipe 3: Cannabis-Infused Raspberry Lemonade

Ingredients:

- 2 cups fresh raspberries
- 1 cup freshly squeezed lemon juice
- 1/2 cup cannabis-infused simple syrup (made with decarboxylated cannabis and a 1:1 mix of water and sugar)
- 2 cups cold water
- Ice cubes
- Fresh mint leaves for garnish

Instructions for Creating Cannabis-Infused Simple Syrup:

- Decarboxylate 7-10 grams of finely powdered cannabis at 220°F (104°C) for 30-45 minutes.
- In a saucepan, add 1 cup of water and 1 cup of sugar.
- Add the decarboxylated cannabis to the mixture and boil on low heat for 2-3 hours, stirring periodically.
- Strain the mixture through a strainer to remove plant detritus and store the infused simple syrup in a jar.

Instructions for Raspberry Lemonade:

- In a blender, purée the fresh raspberries until smooth.
- Strain the raspberry puree through a fine-mesh strainer into a pitcher to remove seeds.
- Add the freshly squeezed lemon juice, cannabis-infused simple syrup, and cold water to the pitcher.
- Stir until completely combined.
- Fill glasses with ice cubes and pour the raspberry lemonade over the ice.
- Garnish with fresh mint leaves for a refreshing touch.

Dosage & Portion:

- Start with one glass of raspberry lemonade containing around 5mg of THC.
- Wait for at least 1 hour before contemplating further intake.
- Adjust the dose in successive batches to fit individual tolerance levels.

Recipe 4: Cannabis-Infused Mango Lassi

Ingredients:

- 1 cup sliced ripe mango
- 1 cup plain yogurt
- 1/2 cup milk of your choice (e.g., almond, soy, or dairy)
- 2 tbsp cannabis-infused honey (made with decarboxylated cannabis and honey)
- 1/4 tsp ground cardamom
- Ice cubes
- Sliced mango and mint leaves for garnish

Instructions for Creating Cannabis-Infused Honey:

- Decarboxylate 7-10 grams of finely powdered cannabis at 220°F (104°C) for 30-45 minutes.
- In a saucepan, slowly cook 1 cup of honey over low heat.
- Add the decarboxylated cannabis to the honey and mix.

- Simmer on low heat for 1-2 hours, stirring periodically.
- Strain the mixture through a strainer to remove plant detritus and store the infused honey in a jar.

Instructions for Mango Lassi:

- In a blender, mix the diced ripe mango, plain yogurt, milk, cannabis-infused honey, and crushed cardamom.
- Blend until smooth and creamy.
- Fill glasses with ice cubes and pour the mango lassi over the ice.
- Garnish with sliced mango and mint leaves for a tropical accent.

Dosage & Portion:

- Start with one glass of mango lassi containing around 5mg of THC.
- Wait for at least 1 hour before contemplating further intake.

- Adjust the dose in successive batches to fit individual tolerance levels.

Recipe 5: Cannabis-Infused Coconut Lime Mojito

Ingredients:

- 1 cup coconut water
- 1/2 cup freshly squeezed lime juice
- 1/4 cup cannabis-infused simple syrup (made with decarboxylated cannabis and a 1:1 mix of water and sugar)
- 1/4 cup fresh mint leaves, plus more for garnish
- 1/4 cup coconut rum (optional for an alcoholic variant)
- Sparkling water
- Ice cubes
- Lime slices for garnish

Instructions for Coconut Lime Mojito:

- In a pitcher, muddle the fresh mint leaves to unleash their flavor.

- Add the coconut water, freshly squeezed lime juice, cannabis-infused simple syrup, and coconut rum (if using) to the pitcher.
- Stir until completely combined.
- Fill glasses with ice cubes and pour the coconut lime mojito over the ice.
- Top with sparkling water for a pleasant zing.
- Garnish with fresh mint leaves and lime slices for a tropical flare.

Dosage & Portion:

- Start with one glass of coconut lime mojito containing around 5mg of THC.
- Wait for at least 1 hour before contemplating further intake.
- Adjust the dose in successive batches to fit individual tolerance levels.

Balanced Ratios Recipes

Recipe 1: Cannabis-Infused Quinoa Veggie Bowl

Ingredients:

- 1 cup cooked quinoa
- 1/2 cup diced cucumber
- 1/2 cup cherry tomatoes, halved
- 1/4 cup chopped red onion
- 1/4 cup crumbled feta cheese
- 2 tbsp cannabis-infused olive oil (made with decarboxylated cannabis and extra virgin olive oil)
- 2 tbsp balsamic vinegar
- Fresh lemon juice
- Salt and black pepper to taste
- Fresh parsley for garnish

Instructions for Creating Cannabis-Infused Olive Oil:

- Decarboxylate 7-10 grams of finely powdered cannabis at 220°F (104°C) for 30-45 minutes.
- In a saucepan, gradually heat 1 cup of extra virgin olive oil over low heat.
- Add the decarboxylated cannabis to the olive oil and mix.
- Simmer on low heat for 2-3 hours, stirring periodically.
- Strain the mixture through a strainer to remove plant detritus and store the infused olive oil in a jar.

Instructions for Quinoa Veggie Bowl:

- In a large bowl, add the cooked quinoa, chopped cucumber, cherry tomatoes, and diced red onion.
- In a separate dish, mix together the cannabis-infused olive oil, balsamic vinegar, fresh lemon juice, salt, and black pepper.

- Drizzle the dressing over the quinoa vegetable mixture and toss until fully covered.
- Sprinkle crumbled feta cheese and fresh parsley over top.
- Serve as a healthful and balanced supper.

Dosage & Portion:

- Start with one serving of quinoa vegetable bowl containing around 5mg of THC.
- Wait for at least 1 hour before contemplating further intake.
- Adjust the dose in successive meals to satisfy individual tolerance levels.

Recipe 2: Cannabis-Infused Grilled Chicken Tacos

Ingredients:

- 2 boneless, skinless chicken breasts
- 2 tbsp cannabis-infused olive oil (made with decarboxylated cannabis and extra virgin olive oil)

- 1 tsp chili powder
- 1/2 tsp cumin
- 1/2 tsp paprika
- Salt and black pepper to taste
- 8 tiny corn tortillas
- Shredded lettuce
- Diced tomatoes
- Diced avocado
- Fresh cilantro for garnish
- Lime wedges for serving

Instructions for Grilled Chicken Tacos:

- In a bowl, combine the cannabis-infused olive oil, chili powder, cumin, paprika, salt, and black pepper to make the marinade.
- Coat the chicken breasts with the marinade and let them marinate for at least 30 minutes.
- Preheat the grill or grill pan over medium-high heat.
- Grill the chicken breasts for 5-6 minutes each side or until thoroughly done.

- Remove the chicken from the grill and let it rest for a few minutes before slicing.
- Heat the corn tortillas on the grill for a few seconds on each side.
- Fill each tortilla with sliced grilled chicken, shredded lettuce, chopped tomatoes, diced avocado, and fresh cilantro.
- Serve the tacos with lime wedges for squeezing.

Dosage & Portion:

- Start with one to two tacos containing roughly 5-10mg of THC.
- Wait for at least 1 hour before contemplating further intake.
- Adjust the dose in successive meals to satisfy individual tolerance levels.

Recipe 3: Cannabis-Infused Mediterranean Quinoa Salad

Ingredients:

- 1 cup cooked quinoa

- 1/2 cup diced cucumber

- 1/2 cup cherry tomatoes, halved

- 1/4 cup chopped red onion

- 1/4 cup crumbled feta cheese

- 2 tbsp cannabis-infused olive oil (made with decarboxylated cannabis and extra virgin olive oil)

- 2 tbsp lemon juice

- 1 tsp dried oregano

- Salt and black pepper to taste

- Kalamata olives for garnish

- Fresh parsley for garnish

Instructions for Mediterranean Quinoa Salad:

- In a large bowl, add the cooked quinoa, chopped cucumber, cherry tomatoes, and diced red onion.

- In a separate dish, mix together the cannabis-infused olive oil, lemon juice, dried oregano, salt, and black pepper.
- Drizzle the dressing over the quinoa salad and stir until fully covered.
- Sprinkle crumbled feta cheese over top and garnish with Kalamata olives and fresh parsley.
- Serve as a refreshing and balanced side dish or light supper.

Dosage & Portion:

- Start with one plate of Mediterranean quinoa salad containing around 5mg of THC.
- Wait for at least 1 hour before contemplating further intake.
- Adjust the dose in successive meals to satisfy individual tolerance levels.

Recipe 4: Cannabis-Infused Salmon and Avocado Sushi Roll

Ingredients:

- 2 nori seaweed sheets
- 1 cup sushi rice, cooked and seasoned with rice vinegar, sugar, and salt
- 4 ounces cooked and cooled salmon, sliced
- 1/2 avocado, thinly sliced
- 2 tbsp cannabis-infused mayonnaise (made with decarboxylated cannabis and store-bought mayonnaise)
- Soy sauce with wasabi for serving

Instructions for Creating Cannabis-Infused Mayonnaise:

- Decarboxylate 7-10 grams of finely powdered cannabis at 220°F (104°C) for 30-45 minutes.
- Mix the decarboxylated cannabis with store-bought mayonnaise until fully mixed.
- Store the cannabis-infused mayonnaise in the refrigerator.

Instructions for Salmon and Avocado Sushi Roll:

1. Lay a bamboo sushi rolling mat on a clean surface and lay a nori seaweed sheet shiny side down on the mat.

2. Wet your hands to avoid sticking, then distribute half of the seasoned sushi rice evenly over the nori, leaving a little border at the top.

3. Arrange half of the sliced salmon and avocado in a line across the middle of the rice.

4. Drizzle the cannabis-infused mayonnaise over the fish and avocado.

5. Carefully pull the edge of the bamboo mat closest to you and start rolling the sushi away from you, pushing gently to secure the filling.

6. Repeat steps 1-5 to construct the second sushi roll.

7. Use a sharp knife to slice each roll into bite-sized pieces.

8. Serve the sushi rolls with soy sauce and wasabi for dipping.

Dosage & Portion:

- Start with one to two sushi rolls containing roughly 5-10mg of THC.
- Wait for at least 1 hour before contemplating further intake.
- Adjust the dose in successive meals to satisfy individual tolerance levels.

Recipe 5: Cannabis-Infused Lentil and Vegetable Curry

Ingredients:

1. 1 cup cooked lentils
2. 1 cup chopped carrots
3. 1 cup chopped bell peppers (mixed colors)
4. 1 cup diced zucchini
5. 1 cup diced eggplant
6. 1 can (14 oz) chopped tomatoes
7. 1 can (14 oz) coconut milk

8. 2 tbsp cannabis-infused olive oil (made with decarboxylated cannabis and extra virgin olive oil)

9. 2 tbsp curry powder

10. 1 tsp ground cumin

11. 1/2 tsp ground turmeric

12. Salt and black pepper to taste

13. Fresh cilantro for garnish

14. Cooked rice or naan bread for serving

Instructions for Lentil and Vegetable Curry:

- In a big saucepan or skillet, heat the cannabis-infused olive oil over medium heat.

- Add the chopped carrots, bell peppers, zucchini, and eggplant to the pan and sauté for a few minutes until slightly softened.

- Stir in the curry powder, powdered cumin, ground turmeric, salt, and black pepper, covering the veggies evenly.

- Pour in the chopped tomatoes (with their juice) and coconut milk, and whisk to blend.

- Simmer the curry mixture for 15-20 minutes until the veggies are soft and the flavors are well mixed.

- Add the cooked lentils to the pan and heat through.

- Serve the lentil and vegetable curry over cooked rice or over naan bread, topped with fresh cilantro.

Dosage & Portion:

- Start with one plate of lentil and vegetable curry containing around 5mg of THC.

- Wait for at least 1 hour before contemplating further intake.

- Adjust the dose in successive meals to satisfy individual tolerance levels.

CHAPTER 4: THE SCIENCE OF MARIJUANA

This chapter discusses the plant's components, the endocannabinoid system, and how edibles interact with human bodies. Gain a greater grasp of the scientific factors underlying the impacts and benefits of cannabis-infused products. Knowledge of these basic concepts will equip you to develop and consume edibles with confidence and responsibly.

The Cannabinoids

Cannabinoids, the chemical components contained in cannabis, play a vital role in influencing the effects of marijuana edibles. The two most well-known cannabinoids are tetrahydrocannabinol (THC) and cannabidiol (CBD). THC is responsible for the psychoactive "high" associated with cannabis ingestion, whereas CBD provides possible medicinal advantages without producing intoxication. Beyond

THC and CBD, the cannabis plant includes over a hundred additional cannabinoids, each with distinct qualities and affects.

For instance, cannabigerol (CBG) shows promise in lowering inflammation, whereas cannabinol (CBN) could benefit in sleep regulation. Understanding the broad diversity of cannabinoids allows for a more educated approach to developing edibles that suit to unique requirements and interests. Accurate dosage and balanced cannabinoid profiles offer a regulated and delightful experience, making marijuana edibles a diverse and individualized alternative for health and relaxation.

How Edibles Differ from Other Cannabis Consumption Methods

Edibles give a different and distinctive experience compared to other cannabis intake techniques. Unlike smoking or vaping, which give quick effects, edibles take longer to kick in as they transit through the digestive system. This delayed onset takes patience, keeping users from overconsumption owing to impatience. Furthermore, edibles deliver a lengthier and more constant impact, making them perfect for sustained comfort and relaxation.

Additionally, edibles reduce the hazards connected with smoking, such as lung difficulties from breathing smoke. They provide a covert solution for cannabis usage, with no detectable aromas or smoke clouds. The vast assortment of food goods accessible, from sweet pleasures to savory delights, appeals to varying taste preferences and nutritional concerns.

However, edibles need exact dose and understanding of individual tolerance levels to minimize possible overconsumption and unwanted consequences. Understanding how edibles vary from other ingestion techniques helps consumers to make educated choices, producing a safer and pleasurable cannabis experience.

Health Benefits and Potential Risks of Cannabis Compounds

Cannabis components, especially cannabinoids like THC and CBD, have been the focus of substantial study into their possible health benefits and accompanying hazards. CBD has showed potential in easing anxiety, lowering inflammation, and assisting with some kinds of epilepsy. It is also being researched for possible help in treating pain and sleeplessness.

THC, on the other hand, has showed usefulness in treating pain, nausea, and muscular spasms, making it helpful for medicinal applications. Both THC and CBD may have neuroprotective qualities and might be effective in treating neurodegenerative illnesses.

However, it's crucial to identify possible hazards linked with cannabis intake. THC may induce cognitive impairment and memory difficulties, and its intoxicating effects might not be acceptable for everyone. Additionally, frequent or excessive use of cannabis, especially with high THC concentration, may lead to dependence and detrimental consequences on mental health.

Understanding the health benefits and possible hazards of cannabis chemicals enables for careful and educated usage, allowing consumers utilize the medicinal capabilities while limiting any negative outcomes. Consultation with healthcare specialists and adherence to precise dose standards play a significant role in maximizing the benefits and limiting dangers connected with cannabis usage.

Current Research and Promising Findings in Medical Cannabis

Medical cannabis research has been slowly improving, offering encouraging discoveries and possible therapeutic uses. Studies have revealed that cannabinoids, especially CBD, may offer promise in treating epilepsy, lowering seizures, and increasing the quality of life for people with some treatment-resistant types of the illness. Additionally, medicinal cannabis is being examined for its potential in reducing chronic pain, multiple sclerosis-related spasticity, and nausea linked with chemotherapy. Researchers are also researching the anti-inflammatory and neuroprotective characteristics of cannabis, indicating potential advantages in treating neurodegenerative illnesses including Alzheimer's and Parkinson's.

Moreover, medicinal cannabis has showed promise in lowering anxiety and symptoms linked with post-traumatic stress disorder (PTSD).

While these results are promising, additional study is required to completely understand the processes and long-term consequences of medicinal cannabis. As the industry continues to expand, medical professionals and policymakers are adopting evidence-based techniques to unlock the full potential of medical cannabis and offer safe, effective therapeutic alternatives for people with varied medical problems.

Chapter 5: Marijuana Politics and Society

In this chapter, I look into the complicated link between marijuana, politics, and society. Explore the historical backdrop of cannabis prohibition, the shifting landscape of legalization, and the societal consequences of changing views towards marijuana. From the war on drugs to the emergence of the cannabis business, we examine how politics and social viewpoints have affected the present status of marijuana usage and regulation.

A Brief History of Marijuana Prohibition and Legalization

Marijuana prohibition stretches back to the early 20th century when many states in the United States started implementing laws banning the use and sale of cannabis. The Marihuana Tax Act of 1937 represented an important federal step towards prohibition, essentially criminalizing marijuana. In the following decades, stringent anti-drug measures were intensified, culminating to the war on drugs in the 1970s.

However, the late 20th and early 21st centuries saw a change in public views towards cannabis. Medical marijuana legalization gained pace, with California leading the movement in 1996. This was followed by a wave of recreational legalization, with Colorado and Washington becoming the first states to allow recreational usage in 2012.

As additional nations followed suit, public opinion on marijuana altered, forcing several countries to adopt progressive legislation. Canada, for instance, legalized recreational marijuana countrywide in 2018.

While marijuana remains illegal at the federal level in the U.S., the rising momentum of state-level legalization and evolving public opinion herald a changing environment for marijuana policy. As society continues to wrestle with the merits and downsides of marijuana usage, the road of prohibition to legalization remains a continuous and difficult narrative.

The Global Landscape: Contrasting Legal Approaches

The worldwide panorama of marijuana legalization reveals a broad assortment of legal systems and attitudes towards cannabis. Some governments retain strong prohibition, implementing heavy penalties for possession and distribution. These governments frequently emphasize drug control laws and see marijuana as a hazardous substance.

Conversely, some nations have adopted a more progressive attitude, embracing varying degrees of legalization. Some have decriminalized possession for personal use, choosing for civil fines rather than criminal proceedings. Others have accepted medical marijuana programs, enabling patients access to cannabis for medicinal reasons. Furthermore, numerous nations have completed full-scale recreational legalization, establishing regulated marketplaces for marijuana goods.

These varied legal methods reflect the intricacies of social norms, public health issues, and economic reasons.

Additionally, they emphasize the continuing arguments concerning the consequences of marijuana usage on people and communities. As additional countries rethink their policies, the global landscape of marijuana legalization remains dynamic, with various nations managing the rewards and pitfalls of adopting diverse legal frameworks.

Public Perception and Changing Attitudes Towards Cannabis

Public view and attitudes towards cannabis have experienced substantial alteration throughout the years. Historically stigmatized and connected with counterculture, marijuana was generally seen unfavorably owing to its illegal status and feared hazards.

However, as medical science evolved and legalization initiatives gained pace, public attitude altered. Increasing evidence of possible medicinal advantages, along with the realization of the failing war on drugs, led to a reassessment of cannabis laws. Advocacy activities, educational endeavors, and media portrayal have had a part in influencing attitudes.

Changing sentiments are mirrored in public opinion surveys indicating increased support for cannabis legalization. Many increasingly consider marijuana as a credible alternative for medicinal treatment and understand its potential economic advantages through the legal cannabis sector.

Despite these good improvements, conflicting perspectives exist, reflecting the continuing social debate concerning cannabis usage and regulation. As education and awareness increase, public opinion will continue to grow, impacting future regulations and societal attitudes towards cannabis.

Social Equity and Criminal Justice Implications

The legalization and regulation of marijuana have attracted attention to the social equity and criminal justice concerns around cannabis. The war on drugs disproportionately affected underprivileged populations, resulting to high rates of arrests and convictions for minor marijuana crimes. As marijuana laws evolve, attempts are being made to remedy these inequalities.

Social equity initiatives attempt to offer possibilities for people and communities harmed by the war on drugs to engage in the legal cannabis sector. These efforts strive to give access to licenses, business help, and expungement of prior convictions.

Moreover, the decriminalization and legalization of marijuana have the potential to alleviate the pressure on criminal justice systems, releasing resources for other vital problems. Additionally, it may enhance police-community relations by shifting law enforcement resources away from low-level marijuana infractions.

However, obstacles persist in attaining genuine social fairness, and certain groups continue to suffer hurdles to entrance into the legal cannabis industry. Advocacy and policy measures are vital to encouraging inclusion and addressing the historical injustices connected to marijuana illegality.

CONCLUSION

The Marijuana Edibles Cookbook digs into the vast and interesting world of cannabis-infused delicacies, giving a full guide to understanding, preparing, and properly consuming these delightful edibles.
From examining the science underlying marijuana and its impact with our bodies to mastering dose, portion management, and infusion methods, this book encourages readers to embark on a voyage of culinary creativity and wellbeing.

Beyond the kitchen, the book dives into the larger panorama of marijuana politics, cultural views, and the pursuit for social equality and justice. As marijuana continues to progress from prohibition to acceptability, the alteration in public opinion and the development of legal frameworks become crucial themes for understanding the future of cannabis in society.

"The Marijuana Edibles Cookbook" advocates responsible use, advocating for educated choices that emphasize safety and well-being. With the counsel offered, readers may enjoy the potential advantages of marijuana edibles while realizing the hazards and being cognizant of individual tolerance levels.

Whether you are a seasoned cannabis fan or a curious novice, this book gives you with information and confidence to go on a culinary journey filled with creativity, healing, and fun. Embrace the art of producing cannabis-infused delights, while being aware, responsible, and appreciative of the ever-changing environment of marijuana.

May your trip with "The Marijuana Edibles Cookbook" be filled with tasty pleasures and a better respect for the dynamic world of cannabis. Happy cooking!

APPRECIATION

Thank you for picking "The Marijuana Edibles Cookbook" as your guide to the world of cannabis-infused delicacies. Your support and interest in this book mean the world to me. I hope you discover inspiration and expertise within these pages to produce tasty delicacies while embracing responsible consumption.

From the science of marijuana to the subtleties of dose and portion management, I intended to give a complete resource for your culinary adventure. As you explore the varied recipes and learn about the social and political backdrop around cannabis, you hope you uncover fresh views and ideas.

Remember, cooking with cannabis is not just about enjoyment but also about attentive and educated decisions. Your dedication to responsible use assures the safety and pleasure of this experience.

Once again, thank you for joining me on this amazing journey. I wish you good cooking and a greater awareness for the fascinating world of cannabis.

Enjoy your culinary creativity and the rewards they provide. pleasant reading and pleasant cooking!

www.ingramcontent.com/pod-product-compliance
Lightning Source LLC
Chambersburg PA
CBHW050042260726
48658CB00005B/1726